The Ultimate Air Fryer Recipe Book

A Full Collection of Easy Recipes for Your Air Fried Meals

Grace Ward

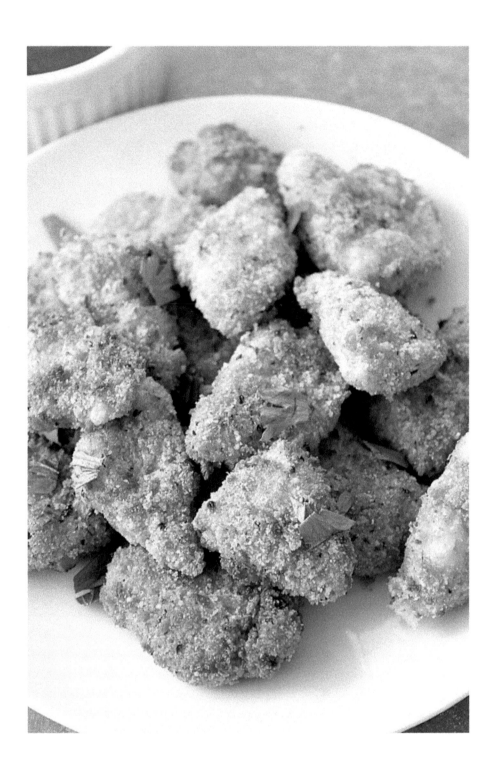

Legal Notice:

Disclaimer Notice:

Please note the information contained within this document is for educational and entertainment purposes only. All effort has been executed to present accurate, up to date, and reliable, complete information. No warranties of any kind are declared or implied. Readers acknowledge that the author is not engaging in the rendering of legal, financial, medical or professional advice. The content within this book has been derived from various sources. Please consult a licensed professional before attempting any techniques outlined in this book.

By reading this document, the reader agrees that under no circumstances is the author responsible for any losses, direct or indirect, which are incurred as a result of the use of information contained within this document, including, but not limited to, — errors, omissions, or inaccuracies.

Table of Contents

Breakfast & Brunch

Bread Rolls With Potato Stuffing
Serves: 4

- Bread - white part only (8 slices)
- Potatoes (5 large)
- Oil - frying and brushing (2 tbsp.)
- Finely chopped coriander (1 small bunch)
- Seeded chopped green chilies (2)
- Turmeric (.5 tsp.)
- Curry leaf sprigs (2)
- Mustard seeds (.5 tsp.)
- Finely chopped small onions (2)
- Salt (as desired)

Directions:

1.Set the Air Fryer at 392° Fahrenheit.

2.Remove the edges of the bread. Peel the potatoes and boil. Mash the potatoes using one teaspoon of salt.

3.On the stovetop, prepare a skillet using one teaspoon of oil. Toss in the mustard seeds and onions. When the seeds sputter, continue frying until they become translucent. Toss in the curry and turmeric.

4.Fry the mixture a few seconds and add the mashed potatoes. Mix well and let it cool. Shape eight portions of dough into an oval shape. Set them aside for now.

5.Wet the bread with water and press it in your palm to remove the excess water. Place the oval potato into the bread and roll it around the potato mixture. Be sure they are completely sealed.

6.Brush the potato rolls with oil and set aside.

7.Set the timer for 12 to 13 minutes. Cook until crispy and browned.

Cheesy Garlic Bread

Serves: 4

- Bread slices
- Round or baguette (5 rounds)
- Sun-dried tomato pesto (5 tsp.)
- Garlic cloves (3)
- Melted butter (4 tbsp.)
- Grated Mozzarella cheese (1 cup)
  Garnish Options:
- Chili flakes
- Chopped basil leaves Oregano

Directions:

1. Set the Air Fryer to reach 356° Fahrenheit.
2. Slice the bread loaf into five thick slices.
3. Spread the butter, pesto, and cheese over the bread.
4. Put the slices in the air Fryer for six to eight minutes.
5. Garnish with your choice of toppings.
6. Note: Round or baguette bread was used for this recipe.

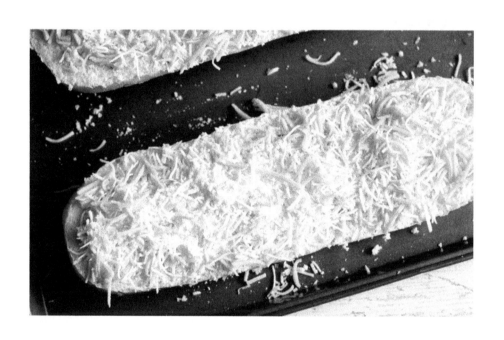

Quick & Easy Poached Eggs

Serves: 4

- Boiling water (3 cups)
- Large egg (1)

Directions:

Set the Air Fryer at 390° Fahrenheit.

Pour boiling water into the Air Fryer basket.

Break the egg into a dish and slide it into the water. Set the basket into the fryer.

Set the timer for 3 minutes. When ready, scoop the poached egg into a plate using a slotted spoon.

Serve with a serving of toast to your liking.

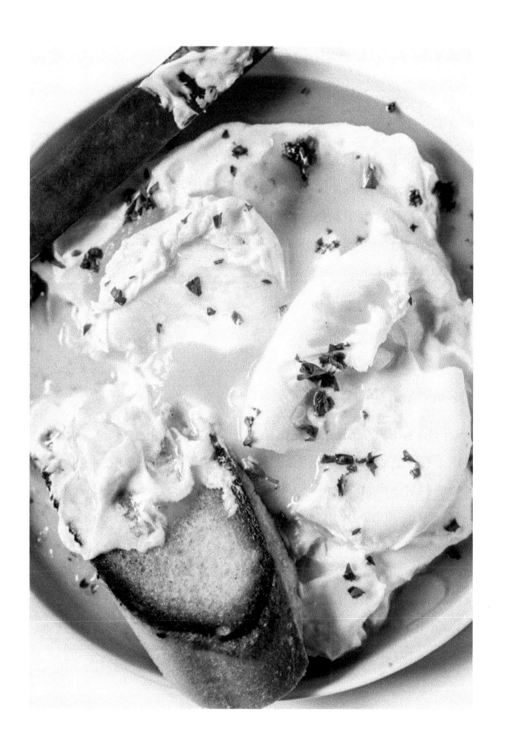

Baked Apple & Walnuts

Serves: 2

- Apple or pear (1 medium)
- Chopped walnuts (2 tbsp.)
- Raisins (2 tbsp.)
- Light margarine (1.5 tsp. - melted)
- Cinnamon (.25 tsp.)
- Nutmeg (.25 tsp.)
- Water (.25 cup)

Directions:

1.Set the Air Fryer temperature at 350° Fahrenheit.

2.Cut the apple/pear in half around the middle and spoon out some of the flesh.

3.Place the apple or pear in the pan (to fit in the Air Fryer).

4.In a small mixing container, combine the cinnamon, nutmeg, margarine, raisins, and walnuts.

5.Add the mixture into the centers of the fruit halves.

6.Pour water into the pan.

7.Air-fry for 20 minutes.

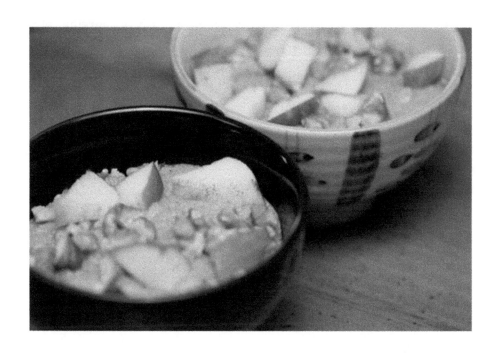

Baked Eggs In A Bread Bowl

Serves: 4

- Large eggs (4)
- Crusty dinner rolls (4)
- Heavy cream (4 tbsp.)
- Mixed herbs - ex. Chopped tarragon, chives, parsley, etc. (4 tbsp.each)
- Grated parmesan cheese (to your liking)

Directions:

1.Set the Air Fryer at 350° Fahrenheit.

2.Use a sharp knife to remove the top of each of the rolls – setting them aside for later. Use a glass or cookie cutter to make a hole in the bread large enough for the egg.

3.Place the rolls in the fryer basket. Break an egg into the roll and top with the cream and herbs. Sprinkle using a portion of the parmesan.

4.Bake for about 20-25 minutes until the egg is set. The bread should be toasted.

5. After 20 minutes, arrange the tops of the bread on the egg and bake a few more minutes to finish the browning process.

6.Remove from the Air Fryer and wait for five minutes. Serve warm.

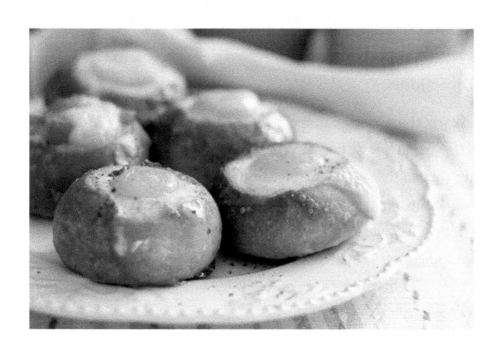

Banana Fritters

Serves: 8

- Vegetable oil (3 tbsp.)
- Breadcrumbs (.75 cup)
- Corn flour (3 tbsp.)
- Ripe peeled bananas (8) Egg white (1)

Directions:

1.Warm the Air Fryer to reach 356° Fahrenheit.

2.Use the low-heat temperature setting to warm a skillet. Pour in the oil and toss in the breadcrumbs. Cook until golden brown.

3.Coat the bananas with the flour. Dip them into the whisked egg white and cover with the breadcrumbs.

4.Arrange the prepared bananas in a single layer of the basket and place thefritter cakes onto a bunch of paper towels to drain before serving.

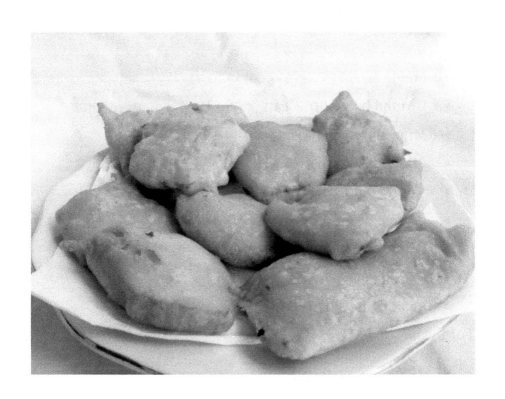

Lunch & Dinner

Bourbon Bacon Burger

Servings Provided: 2

- Bourbon (1 tbsp.)
- Brown sugar (2 tbsp.)
- Maple bacon (3 strips - cut in half)
- Ground beef - 80% lean (.75 lb.)
- Minced onion (1 tbsp.)
- BBQ sauce (2 tbsp.)
- Salt (.5 tsp.)
- Freshly ground black pepper (as desired)
- Colby Jack/Monterey Jack (2 slices)
- Kaiser rolls (2)
- LETTUCE AND TOMATO

For the Sauce:

- BBQ sauce (2 tbsp.)
- Mayonnaise (2 tbsp.)
- Ground paprika (.25 tsp.)

Directions:

Warm the Air Fryer at 390° Fahrenheit and pour a little water into the bottom of the fryer drawer.   Combine the brown sugar and bourbon in a small bowl. Place the bacon strips in the fryer basket and brush with the brown sugar mixture. Air-fry for four minutes. Flip the bacon over, and recoat using more brown sugar and air- fry for another 4 minutes until crispy. Prepare the burgers. Combine the onion, ground beef, barbecue sauce, salt, and pepper in a large bowl. Shape the meat into two burgers. Place the burgers in the Air Fryer basket and cook them at 370° Fahrenheit for 15-20 minutes (15 minutes for rare to medium-rare or 20 minutes for well-done). Flip the burgers halfway through the cooking process.

Prepare the burger sauce by combining the BBQ sauce, mayonnaise, paprika, and freshly ground black pepper in a bowl. When the burgers are finished to your taste, add a slice of Colby Jack cheese to each patty and air-fry for another minute, or until the cheese has melted. (To keep the cheese slice from blowing off in your air fryer, pin it to the burger with a toothpick.) On the inside of the Kaiser rolls, spread the sauce, then top with the burgers, bourbon bacon, lettuce, and tomato, and serve.

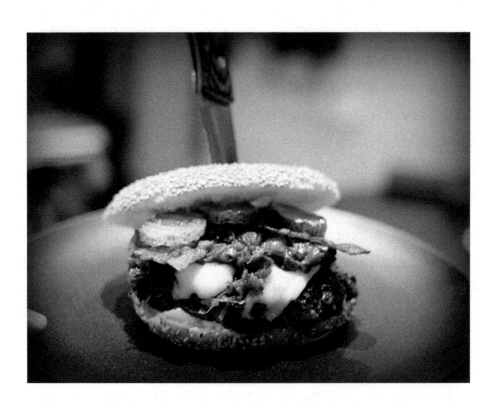

Egg Rolls

Servings Provided: 16

- Frozen corn (2 cups)
- Black beans (15 oz. can)
- Spinach (13.5 oz. can)
- Jalapeno Jack cheese (1.5 cups)
- Sharp cheddar cheese (1 cup)
- Diced green chiles (4 oz. can)
- Green onions (4)
- Scallions/Green onions (1 bunch)
- Salt (1 tsp.)
- Ground cumin (1 tsp.)
- Chili powder (1 tsp.)
- Egg roll wrappers (16 oz. pkg.)

Directions:

Preheat the Air Fryer to 390° Fahrenheit. Do the prep. Drain and rinse the beans. Drain the chiles and spinach. Shred the cheese and slice the onions. Thaw and mix in a large bowl the corn, beans, spinach, both types of cheese, salt, green chiles, green onions, cumin, and chili powder .

An egg roll wrapper should be put at an angle. Lightly moisten all four edges with water. In the center of the wrapper, place around 1/4 cup of the filling. To make a roll, fold one corner over the filling and tuck in the ends. Repeat with the remaining wrappers and a light mist of cooking spray for each egg roll. Arrange the egg rolls in the basket, making sure they are not touching, cooking in batches if necessary. Cook for 8 minutes on one hand, then flip and cook until the skins are crispy (4 min.).

Air Bread & Egg Butter

Serves: 19

- Eggs (3)
- Baking powder (1 tsp.)
- Sea salt (.25 tsp.)
- Almond flour (1 cup)
- Unchilled butter (.25 cup)

Directions:

1 Set the Air Fryer at 350° Fahrenheit.

2 Whisk the eggs with a hand mixer. Mix in the rest of the fixings to make a dough. Knead the dough and cover using a tea towel for about ten minutes.

3 Air-fry the bread 15 minutes. Remove the bread and let it cool down on a wooden board.

4 Slice and serve with your favorite meal or as it is with butter (below).

For The Butter:

Serves: 4

- Eggs (4)

- Salt (1 tsp.)
- Butter (4 tbsp.)

Directions:

1 Prepare the Air Fryer basket using a layer of foil and add the eggs.

2 Air-fry the eggs at 320° Fahrenheit for 17 minutes. Transfer to an ice- cold water bath to chill.

3 Peel and chop the eggs and combine with the rest of the fixings. Enjoy with your Air Fried Bread.

Hawaiian Pizzas

Servings Provided: 12

- Thomas' Light Multi-Grain English Muffins (1 pkg.)
- Pizza sauce (1 cup)
- Canadian Bacon (.5 cup)
- Crushed pineapple (.25 cup)
- Shredded mozzarella cheese (1-2 cups)

Directions:

Set the fryer at 355° Fahrenheit. Separate the English muffins gently with your finger. Make sure the air can still circulate inside the Air Fryer by placing a sheet of foil inside. Using a nonstick cooking spray, coat it.Place the English muffin halves in the fryer (as many as can fit neatly). Sauce, Canadian bacon, pineapple, and shredded cheese go on top of each half. Air-fry for 5 minutes. It's essential to check them after about 3 minutes to be sure all toppings are still cooking evenly. Remove and serve.

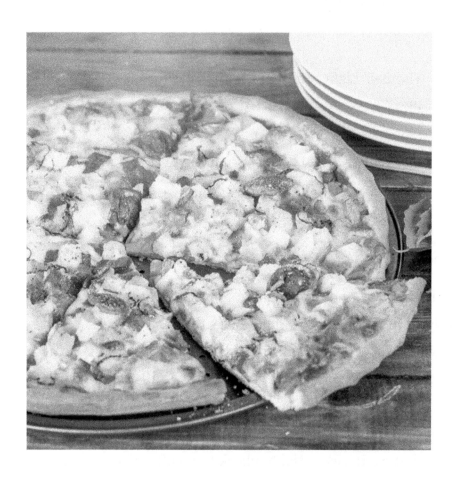

Vegetable Egg Rolls

Preparation time: 15 minutes **Cooking time**: 10 minutes
Servings: 8 egg rolls

- ½ cup chopped mushrooms
- ½ cup grated carrots
- ½ cup chopped zucchini
- 2 green onions, chopped
- 1 tablespoons low-Sodium soy sauce
- 8 egg roll wrappers
- 1 tablespoon cornstarch
- 1 egg, beaten

Directions:

Stir together the mushrooms, carrots, zucchini, green onions, and soy sauce in a medium mixing dish. On a work surface, spread out the egg roll wrappers. On top of each, place 3 tablespoons of the vegetable mixture. Combine the cornstarch and egg in a small bowl and whisk well. Clean the egg roll wrappers' edges with some of this mixture. Wrap the wrappers around the vegetable filling and roll them up. To seal the egg rolls, brush some of the egg mixture on the outside. Cook for 7–10 minutes in the air fryer, or until the egg rolls are brown and crunchy.

NUTRITION: Calories: 112; total Fat: 1g; saturated Fat: 0g; Cholesterol: 23mg; Sodium: 417mg; Carbohydrates: 21g; Fiber: 1g; Protein: 4g

Black Peppercorns Meatloaf

Servings Provided: 4

- Parsley (1 tbsp.)
- Oregano (1 tbsp.)
- Basil (1 tbsp.)
- Salt and pepper (to your liking)
- Ground beef (4.5 lb.)
- Large onion (1 diced)
- Worcestershire sauce (1 tsp.)
- Tomato ketchup (3 tbsp.)
- Breadcrumbs (1 slice of bread if homemade)

Directions:

Set the temperature setting at 356° Fahrenheit.

Toss the beef, herbs, onion, Worcestershire sauce, and ketchup together and mix well (5 min.). Mix in the breadcrumbs. Scoop the meatloaf into the baking dish and arrange it in the Air Fryer basket. Air-fry for 25 minutes.

Coconut Red Lentil Curry

Preparation time: 5 mins **Cooking time**: 13 mins.
Servings: 6

- ½ teaspoon of turmeric powder
- 3 tablespoons of fresh ginger, grated
- 3 cups of tomatoes, diced
- ½ cup of cilantro
- 3 teaspoons of salt
- 1 cup of red kidney beans, boiled
- 1½ cups of black gram beans, boiled
- 2 tablespoons of water
- 2 tablespoons of oil
- 2 teaspoons of cumin seeds
- 1 cup of onions, finely diced
- 3 teaspoons of red chili powder
- 2 teaspoons of garam masala
- 2 cups of coconut cream

Directions:

Set the instant vortex on roast to 375 degrees f for 10 minutes. Sauté onions and cumin seeds in the olive oil in a pan for about 3 minutes. Stir in the tomatoes, ginger, turmeric powder, beans, salt, water, and red chili powder. Transfer this mixture into the

Cooking dish and place on the Cooking tray. Insert the Cooking tray in the vortex when it displays "add food". Remove from the vortex when Cooking time is complete. Serve warm.

NUTRITION: Calories: 422 Protein: 13.4g Carbs : 43.6g Fat: 12.6g

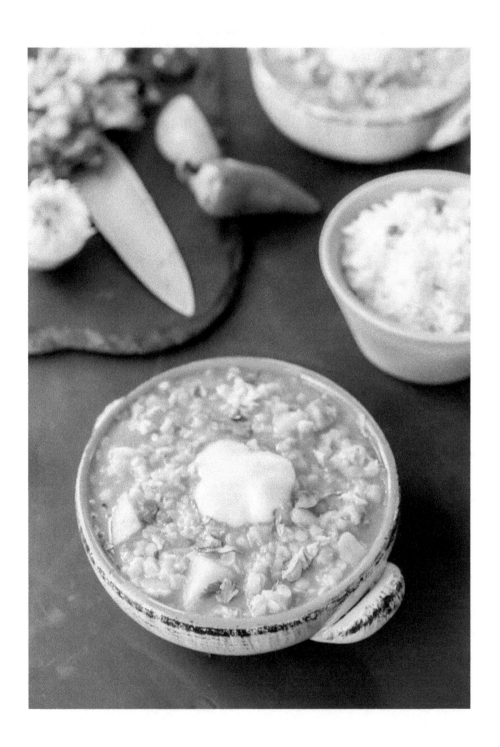

Saffron Cream Cheese Rice

Preparation time: 10 mins **Cooking time:** 15 mins
Servings: 4

- 3 garlic cloves, minced
- 1 cup of white wine
- 3 tablespoons of hot vegetable broth
- 2 cups of rice, boiled
- 3 tablespoons of olive oil
- 1 cup of onions, finely chopped
- 8 oz. Of soft cream cheese
- ½ cup of pecans, coarsely chopped
- Salt and black pepper, to taste
- 1 teaspoon of saffron threads, dissolved in warm water
- 1 tablespoons of fresh lemon juice

Directions:

Set the instant vortex on roast to 375 degrees f for 12 minutes. Sauté onions and garlic in the olive oil in a pan for about 3 minutes. Stir in rest of the Ingredients except cream cheese and lemon juice. Transfer this mixture into the Cooking dish and place on the Cooking tray. Insert the Cooking tray in the vortex when it displays "add food". Remove from the vortex when cooking time is complete. Squeeze with lemon juice and top with cream cheese to serve.

NUTRITION: Calories: 575 Protein: 13.4g Carbs : 43.6g Fat: 12.6g

Sunny Lentils

Preparation time: 10 mins **Cooking time**: 12 mins
Servings: 4

- 1/3 cup of red bell pepper, chopped
- ½ teaspoon of dried tarragon
- 1 cup of tomatoes, diced
- 3 tablespoons of sweetened coconut, shredded
- ¼ teaspoon of curry powder
- ¼ cup of water
- Salt and black pepper, to taste
- 1 cup of red lentils, boiled
- 1 tablespoon of olive oil
- 1/3 cup of green bell pepper, chopped
- 1 tablespoon of garlic, minced
- 1/3 cup of onions, chopped

Directions:

Set the instant vortex on roast to 375 degrees f for 8 minutes. Sauté onions, garlic, green bell pepper, red bell pepper, tarragon, and spices in the olive oil in a pan for about 4 minutes. Stir in the tomatoes, red lentils, and coconut. Transfer this mixture into the Cooking dish and place on the Cooking tray. Insert the Cooking tray in the vortex when it displays "add food". Remove from the vortex when Cooking time is complete. Serve warm.

NUTRITION: Calories: 235 Protein: 13.4g Carbs : 43.6g Fat: 12.6g

Kale Rice

Preparation time: 10 mins **Cooking time**: 20 mins.
Servings: 4

- ¼ cup of white wine
- 1 tablespoons of vegetable stock
- 2 tablespoons of basil, chopped
- ½ cup of parmesan, grated
- 1½ cups of rice, boiled
- 1 bunch kale leaves, chopped and stems removed
- 1 cup of onions, finely chopped
- 2 garlic cloves, minced
- ½ teaspoon of salt
- ½ teaspoon of black pepper
- ½ teaspoon of red pepper flakes
- 2 tablespoons of apple cider vinegar
- 2 tablespoons of olive oil

Directions:

Set the instant vortex on air fryer to 375 degrees f for 12 minutes. Sauté onions and garlic in the olive oil in a pan for about 3 minutes. Stir in the rice, wine and vegetable broth. Transfer this mixture into the Cooking dish and place on the Cooking tray. Insert the Cooking tray in the vortex when it displays "add food". Remove from the vortex when Cooking time is complete. Stir in the kale leaves, chopped herbs, apple cider vinegar, salt, black pepper, cheese, and red pepper flakes. Cook again in the vortex for about 5 minutes and dish out to serve warm.

NUTRITION: Calories: 307 Protein: 13.4g Carbs : 43.6g Fat: 12.6g

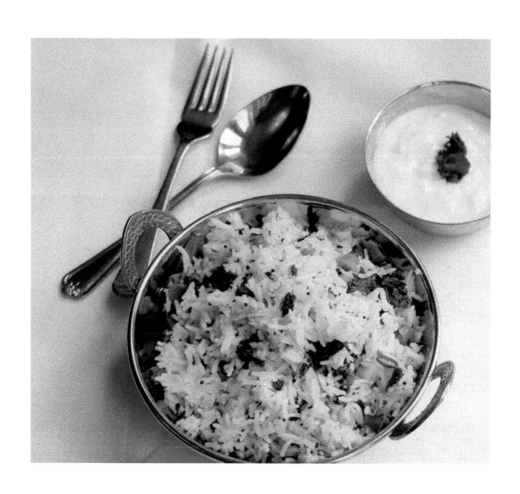

Zucchini Cakes

Preparation time: 20 minutes **Cooking time**: 30 minutes
Servings: 12

- 3 cups zucchini
- ½ cup finely chopped onion
- ¼ tsp oregano
- ¼ tsp black pepper
- ½ tsp salt
- Dash of garlic powder
- 2 tbsp parsley, finely chopped
- ½ cup grated parmesan cheese
- ¼ cup vegetable oil
- 4 eggs, lightly beaten

Directions:

Preheat the oven to 350 degrees Fahrenheit. Using cooking oil, gently coat a baking dish. Stir together all of the mentioned ingredients in a large mixing bowl until well mixed. Pour the ingredients into the baking dish and spread them out evenly. Preheat the oven to 350 degrees Fahrenheit and bake for 30 minutes or until lightly browned. Break the cake into 12 squares.

NUTRITION: Carbs: 9g Fat: 8g Protein: 5g Fiber: 0g Sodium: 161mg

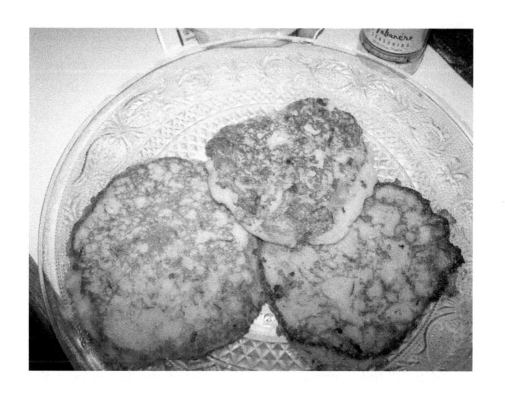

Peanut Butter Cubes

Preparation time: 20 minutes **Cooking time**: 20 minutes
Servings: 20

- 1 cup of peanut butter
- 2 tsp of vanilla extract
- 1 cup of peanuts
- 5 cups of cheerios cereal
- 1/2 cup of white Sugar
- 1/2 cup of corn syrup
- 1 scoop of vanilla powder
- 4 tbsp of mini chocolate chips

Directions:

Combine white sugar and light corn syrup in a medium saucepan. Get the water to a boil. Combine the peanut butter, vanilla, and protein powder in a mixing bowl.

Blend until fully smooth. In a big mixing bowl, combine the peanut butter, cheerios, and peanuts. Over the cheerios and peanuts, pour the peanut butter mixture. Stir until it is well blended. Spread the cheerio mixture in a baking dish that has been greased with nonstick cooking spray.

Cook for 20 mins in fryer.

NUTRITION: Carbs : 19g Fat: 7g Protein: 5g Fiber: 1.5g Sodium: 70mg

Roasted Vegetables

Preparation time: 20 minutes **Cooking time**: 25 minutes
Servings: 6

- 3 oz raw broccoli florets
- 7 oz raw cauliflower florets
- 8 oz raw yellow summer squash
- 8 oz raw zucchini
- 7 oz raw carrots
- oz raw red onion
- 2 tbsp olive oil
- 2 tbsp balsamic vinegar
- Salt, to taste

Directions:

Preheat the oven to 425 degrees Fahrenheit. Set aside a baking sheet lightly coated with Cooking spray. Combine all of the vegetables in a big mixing bowl and stir to combine. After drizzling the olive oil and vinegar over the vegetables, season them with salt and pepper. To layer evenly, toss. On the prepared baking sheet, roast the vegetables for about 25 minutes, or until they are caramelized.

NUTRITION: Carbs: 11g Fat: 6g Protein: 3g Fiber: 4g Sodium: 35.5mg

Air Fried Beef & Potato

Serves: 4

- Mashed potatoes (3 cups)
- Ground beef (1 lb.)
- Eggs (2)
- Garlic powder (2 tbsp.)
- Sour cream (1 cup)
- Freshly cracked black pepper (as desired)
- Salt (1 pinch)

Directions:

1. Set the Air Fryer to reach 390° Fahrenheit.

2. Combine all of the fixings in a mixing container.

3. Scoop it into a heat-safe dish.

4. Arrange in the fryer to cook for two minutes.

5. Serve for lunch or a quick dinner.

Beef & Bacon Taco Rolls

Serves: 2

- Ground beef (2 cups)
- Bacon bits (.5 cup)
- Tomato salsa (1 cup)
- Shredded Monterey Jack Cheese (1 cup)

As desired - with the beef taco spices:

- Garlic powder Chili powder Black pepper
- Turmeric coconut wraps/your choice (4)

Directions:

1.Warm the Air Fryer to reach 390° Fahrenheit.

2.Mix the beef and chosen spices, and add it to each of the fixings into the wraps.

3.Roll up the wraps and arrange them in the Air Fryer.

4.Set the timer for 15 minutes and serve.

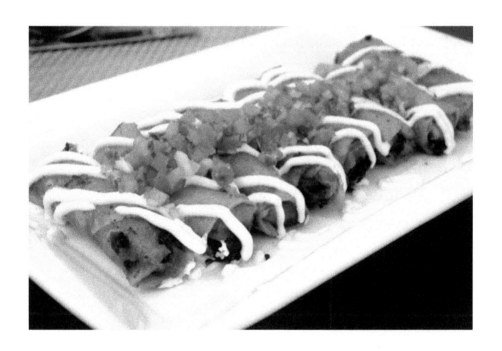

Beef Empanadas

Serves: 4

- Onion (1 small)
- Cloves of garlic (2)
- Olive oil (1 tbsp.)
- Ground beef (1 lb.)
- Empanada shells (1 pkg.)
- Green pepper (.5 of 1)
- Cumin (.5 tsp.)
- Tomato salsa (.25 cup)
- Egg yolk (1)
- Pepper and sea salt (to your liking)

Directions:

1.Peel and mince the garlic and onion. Deseed and dice the pepper.

2.Pour the oil to a skillet using the high-heat temperature setting.

3.Fry the ground beef until browned. Drain the grease and add the onions and garlic. Cook for 4 minutes. Combine the remainder of fixings (omitting the milk, egg, and shells for now). Cook using the low setting for 10 minutes.

4.Make an egg wash with the yolk and milk.

5.Add the meat to half of the rolled dough, brushing the edges with the wash. Fold it over and seal using a fork, brushing with the wash, and adding it to the basket.

6.Continue the process until all are done. Set the timer for 10 minutes in the Air Fryer at 350° Fahrenheit. Serve.

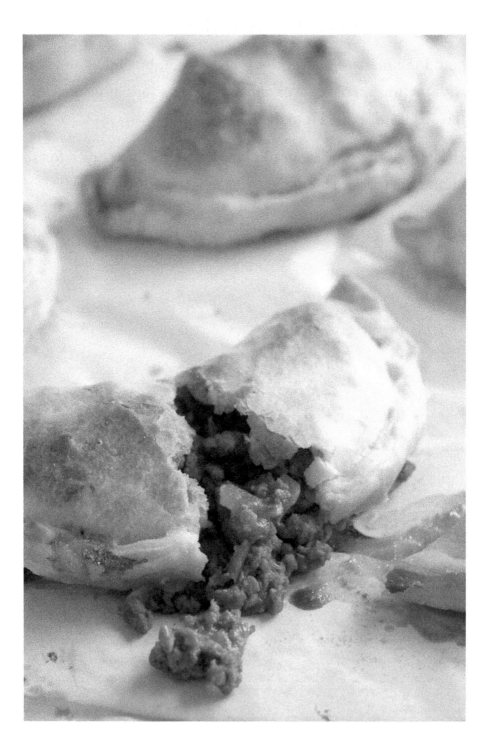

Beef Stew

Serves: 6

- Butter (2 tsp.)
- Beef short ribs (10 oz.)
- Salt (.25 tsp.)
- Turmeric (1 tsp.)
- Chili flakes (.5 tsp.)
- Green pepper (1)
- Kale (4 oz.)
- Chicken stock (1 cup)
- Onion (half of 1)
- Green peas (4 oz.)

Directions:

1.Heat the Air Fryer at 360° Fahrenheit.

2.Measure the two teaspoons of butter to melt in the fryer basket. Add the ribs. Sprinkle with the salt, turmeric, and chili flakes. Set the timer to air- fry for 15 minutes.

3.Remove the seeds and chop the kale and green pepper. Dice the onion.

4.When the timer buzzes, pour in the stock, peppers, onions, peas, and the peeled garlic clove.

5.Stir well and add the chopped kale. Set the timer for eight more minutes before serving.

Asparagus Omelet

Serves: Eggs (3)

- Pepper & salt (1 pinch each)
- Steamed asparagus tips (5)
- Warm water (2 tbsp.)
- Parmesan cheese (1 tbsp.)

Directions:

1. Set the Air Fryer temperature setting to 320° Fahrenheit.
2. Whisk the eggs, water, pepper, salt, and cheese.
3. Spritz a skillet with cooking oil spray and steam the asparagus.
4. Add to the fryer basket. Pour in the egg mixture.
5. Fry for 5 minutes and serve.

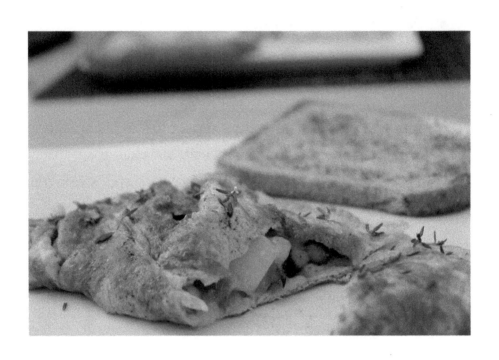

Bacon Egg & Cheese Roll-Ups

Serves: 4

- Unsalted butter (2 tbsp.)
- Chopped onion (.25 cup)
- Almond flour (1 cup)
- Medium green bell pepper (half of 1)
- Large eggs (6)
- Shredded sharp cheddar cheese (1 cup)
- Sugar-free bacon (12 slices)
- For Dipping: Mild salsa (.5 cup)

Directions:

1 Prepare a skillet using the medium heat temperature setting to melt butter.

2 Discard the seeds and dice the peppers and onion. Toss them into the pan and sauté for three minutes.

3 Whisk the eggs in another small mixing bowl, and pour into the pan. Scramble the eggs with the onions and peppers about five minutes or until fluffy and fully cooked. Take it away from the heat and set aside.

4 Heat the Air Fryer to reach 350° Fahrenheit.

5 Arrange three slices of bacon side by side. You can overlap them about 1/4-inch. Divide the eggs in a pile (on the side that's the closest to you). Garnish the top of the eggs with a portion of cheese.

6 Roll the bacon tightly around the eggs. Hold them together using a toothpick or skewer if necessary. Arrange each of the rolls into the Air Fryer basket.

7 Air-fry them for 15 minutes. Turn the rolls halfway through the cooking time.

8 The bacon will be browned and crispy when done.

9 Serve immediately with salsa for dipping. It's great for brunch!

Black Peppercorns Meatloaf

Serves: 4

- Parsley (1 tbsp.)
- Oregano (1 tbsp.)
- Basil (1 tbsp.)
- Salt and pepper (to your liking)
- Ground beef (4.5 lb.)
- Large onion (1 diced)
- Worcestershire sauce (1 tsp.)
- Tomato ketchup (3 tbsp.)
- Breadcrumbs (1 slice of bread if homemade)

Directions:

1.Set the temperature setting at 356° Fahrenheit.

2.Toss the beef, herbs, onion, Worcestershire sauce, and ketchup together and mix well (5 min.). Mix in the breadcrumbs.

3.Scoop the meatloaf into the baking dish and arrange it in the Air Fryer basket. Air-fry for 25 minutes.

Breaded Beef Schnitzel

Serves: 1

- Olive oil (2 tbsp.)
- Thin beef schnitzel (1)
- Gluten-free breadcrumbs (.5 cup)
- Egg (1)

Directions:

1.Heat the Air Fryer a couple of minutes (356° Fahrenheit).

2.Combine the breadcrumbs and oil in a shallow bowl. Whisk the egg in another mixing container.

3.Dip the beef into the egg, and then the breadcrumbs.
4.Arrange in the basket of the Air Fryer.

5.Air-fry 12 minutes and serve.

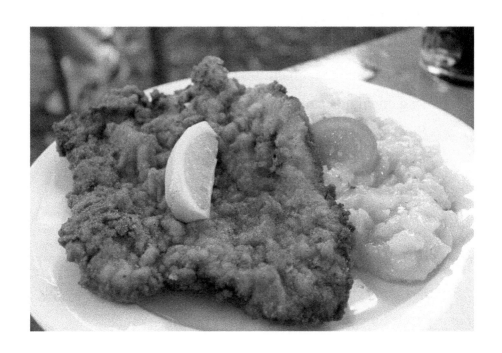

Cheesy Beef Enchiladas

Serves: 4

- Ground beef (1 lb.)
- Regular/Gluten-free taco seasoning (1 pkg.)
- Gluten-free tortillas (8)
- Black beans (1 can)
- Diced tomatoes (1 can)
- Mild chopped green chilies (1 can)
- Red enchilada sauce (1 can)
- Shredded Mexican Cheese (1 cup)
- Chopped fresh cilantro (1 cup)
- Sour cream (.5 cup)

Directions:

1.Set the Air Fryer temperature ahead of cooking time at 355° Fahrenheit. Line the fryer with a layer of foil if you choose.

2.Drain and rinse the beans. Drain the tomatoes and chiles.

3.Brown the ground beef in a skillet. Add in the taco seasoning.

4.Prepare four tortillas by adding beans, tomatoes, beef, and chilies.

5.Arrange the prepared tortillas in the basket of the Air Fryer.

6.After they are prepared, pour the enchilada sauce evenly over them, and garnish using the cheese.

7.Cook for five minutes in the Air Fryer.

8.Carefully remove, add the desired toppings, and serve.

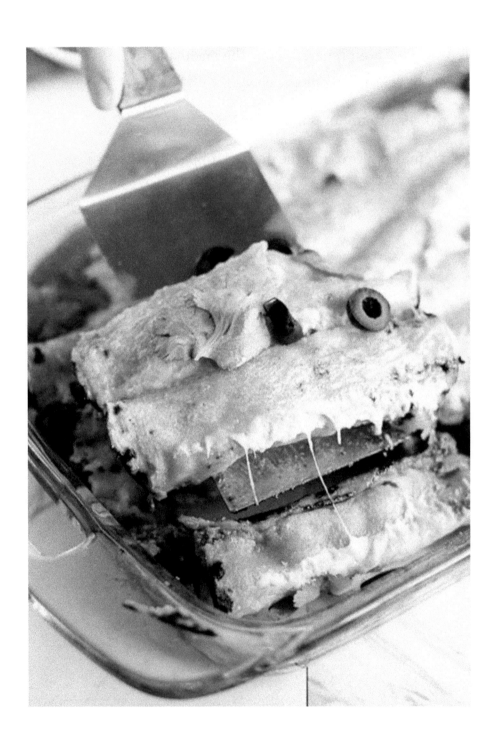

Side Dishes

Charred Shishito Peppers

Servings Provided: 4

- Olive oil (1 tsp.)
- Juiced lemon (1)
- Shishito peppers (20)
- Sea salt (to taste)

Directions:

Set the Air Fryer at 390° Fahrenheit. Toss the peppers in with the oil and salt. Add them to the basket and air-fry for five minutes. Serve with a squeeze of lemon on a platter.

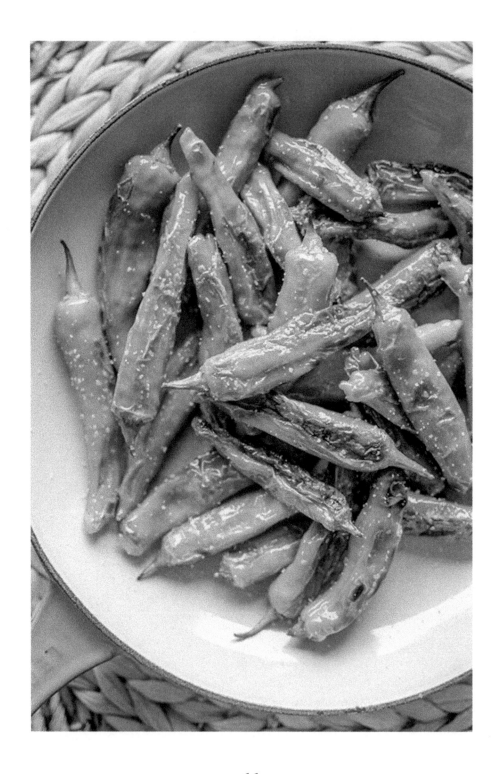

Air-Fried Okra

Serves: 4

- All-purpose flour (.25 cup)
- Cornmeal (1 cup)
- Large egg (1)
- Okra pods (.5 lb)
- Salt (as desired)

Directions:

1.Set the Air Fryer to 400° Fahrenheit.

2.Whisk the egg in a shallow dish. Slice and stir in the okra.

3.Mix the cornmeal and flour in a gallon-size zipper plastic bag. Drop five slices of okra into the cornmeal mixture, zip the bag, and shake. Remove the breaded okra to a plate. Repeat with remaining okra slices.

4.Place half of the breaded slices into the fryer basket and mist using the cooking spray. Set the timer for four minutes. Shake the basket and mist okra with cooking oil spray again. Cook another four minutes. Shake the basket one last time and cook for another two minutes. Remove the okra from the basket and salt to your liking.

5.Repeat with the remaining okra slices.

Avocado & Bacon Fries

Serves: 2

- Egg (1)
- Almond flour (1 cup)
- Bacon – cooked – small bits (4 strips)
- Avocados (2 large)
- For Frying: Olive oil

Directions:

1.Set the Air Fryer at 355° Fahrenheit.

2.Whisk the eggs in one container. Add the flour with the bacon in another.

3.Slice the avocado using lengthwise cuts. Dip into the eggs, then the flour mixture.

4.Drizzle oil in the fryer tray and cook for 10 minutes on each side or until they're the way you like them.

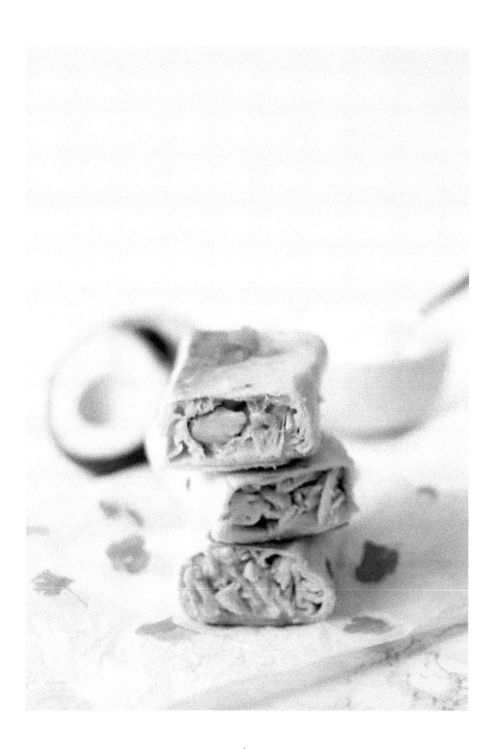

Battered Baby Ears Of Corn

Serves: 4

- Carom seeds (.5 tsp.)
- Almond flour (1 cup)
- Chili powder (.25 tsp.)
- Garlic powder (1 tsp.)
- Boiled baby ears of corn (4)
- Baking soda (1 pinch)
- Salt (to your liking)

Directions:

1.Warm the Air Fryer to reach 350° Fahrenheit.

2.Whisk the flour, salt, garlic powder, baking soda, chili powder, and carom seeds. Pour a little water into a bowl to make a batter. Dip the boiled corn in the mixture and arrange it in a foil-lined fryer basket. Set the timer for 10 minutes.

3.Serve with your favorite entrée.

Breaded Avocado Fries

- Servings Provided: 2 :
- Large avocado (1)
- Breadcrumbs (.5 cup)
- Egg (1)
- Salt (.5 tsp.)

Directions:

1.Warm the Air Fryer to reach 390° Fahrenheit.

2.Peel, remove the pit, and slice the avocado.

3.Prepare two shallow dishes, one with the breadcrumbs and salt, and one with a whisked egg.

4.Dip the avocado into the egg – then the breadcrumbs.

5.Add to the Air Fryer for ten minutes.

6.Serve as a side dish or an appetizer.

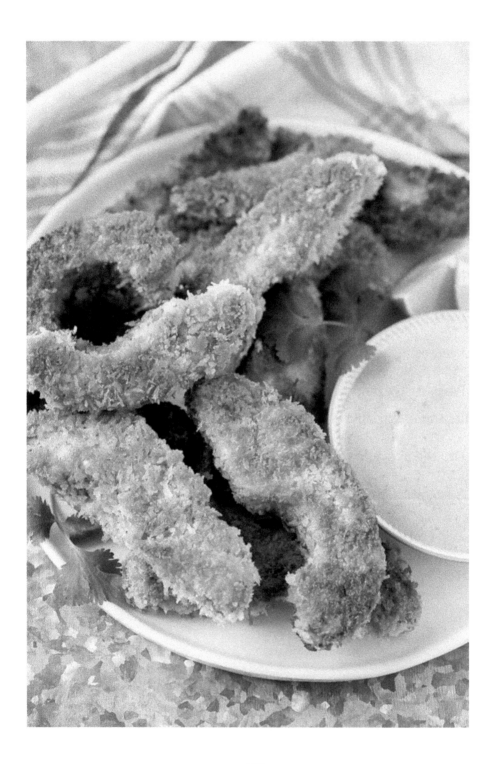

Brussels Sprouts

Serves: 4-5

- Olive oil (5 tbsp.)
- Fresh brussels sprouts (1 lb.)
- Kosher salt (.5 tsp.)

Directions:

1.Prep the vegetables. Trim the stems and discard any damaged outer leaves. Cut into halves, rinse, and pat dry. Toss with the oil and salt.

2.Set the fryer temperature ahead of time to 390° Fahrenheit.

3.Toss the sprouts into the basket and air-fry for 15 minutes.

4.Shake the basket to ensure even browning.

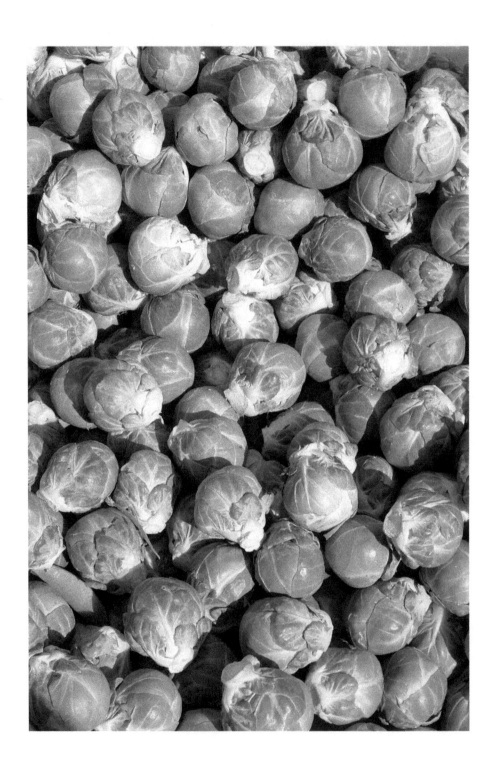

Buffalo Cauliflower

Serves: 4

- Breadcrumbs (1 cup)
- Cauliflower florets (4 cups)
- Buffalo sauce (.25 cup)
- Melted butter (.25 cup)

Directions:

1.Melt the butter in a microwaveable dish. Whisk in the buffalo sauce.

2.Dip the florets in the butter mixture. Use the stem as a handle, holding it over a cup and let the excess drip away.

3.Dredge the florets through the breadcrumbs. Drop them into the Air Fryer. Set the timer for 14 to 17 minutes at 350° Fahrenheit. (The unit will not need to preheat since it is calculated into the time.)

4.Shake the basket several times during the cooking process. Serve alongside your favorite dip, making sure to eat it right away because the crunchiness goes away quickly.

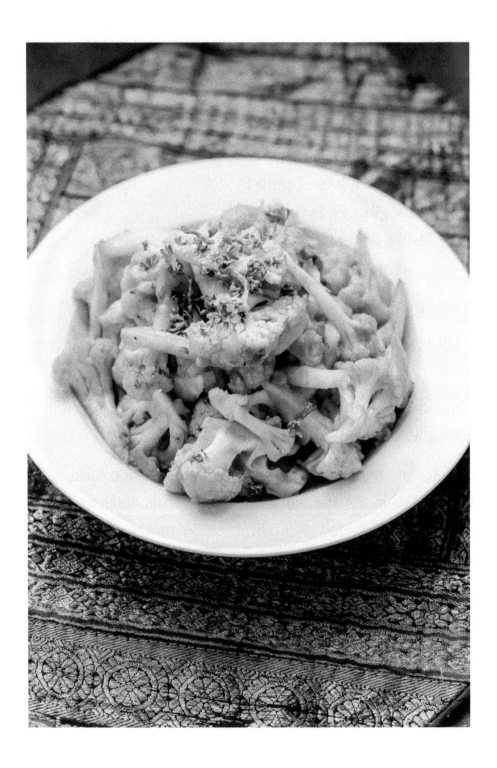

Buttery Blossoming Onions

Serves: 4

- Small onions (4)
- Dollops of butter (4)
- Olive oil (1 tbsp.)

Directions:

1.Preheat the Air Fryer to reach 350º Fahrenheit.

2.Peel the skin from the onion and remove the top and bottom to create flat ends.

3.Soak the onions in salted water for four (4) hours to remove its harshness.

4.Slice the onion as far down as you can without severing its body. Cut four times - making eight segments.

5.Toss the prepared onions into the fryer basket. Drizzle with oil, adding a dollop of butter to each one.

6.Cook in the fryer until the outside is dark (30 minutes).

7.Note: Four dollops equals about four (4) heaping tablespoons.

Crispy Onion Rings

Servings Provided: 2:

- Coconut flour (2 tbsp.)
- Grated parmesan cheese (2 tbsp.)
- Egg (1)
- Large onion (1 in ringlets)
- Garlic powder (1 pinch)
- Pepper and salt (as desired)
- Olive oil (.25 cup)

Directions:

1. Whisk the flour, spices, and grated cheese.
2. Set the Air Fryer at 400° Fahrenheit.
3. Whisk the eggs in a separate mixing container and add the onion rings. Soak a minute or so, and dip into the flour mixture.
4. Place in the Air Fryer basket, setting the timer for 6 minutes per side.
5. Serve as a quick snack or favorite side dish.

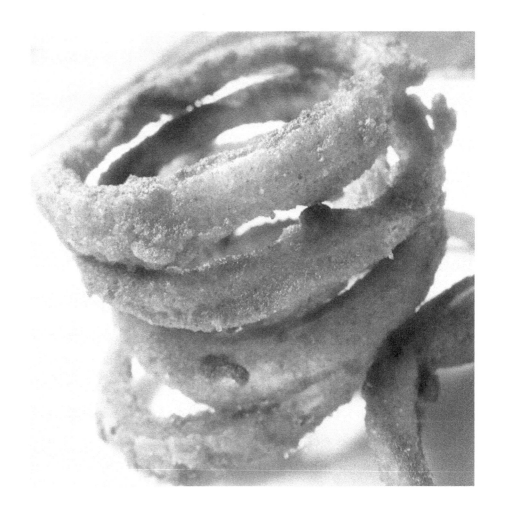

Plant-Based Recipes

Air Fried Kale Chips

Preparation time: 5 minutes **Cooking time:** 10 minutes **Servings**: 6

- ¼ tsp. Himalayan salt
- 3 tbsp. Yeast Avocado oil
- 1 bunch of kale

Directions:

Clean the kale by rinsing it and patting it dry with paper towels. Tear the leaves of the kale into big chunks. Mind that they can shrink when they cook, so use big bits. In a cup, spritz the kale parts with avocado oil until they are shiny. To taste, season with a pinch of salt and a pinch of yeast. Toss the kale leaves together with your fingertips. Set the temperature to 350°F and pour half of the kale mixture into the air fryer basket, and set time to 5 minutes.

NUTRITION: Calories: 55 Cal Total Fat: 10 g Saturated Fat: 0 g Cholesterol: 0 mg Sodium: 0 mg Total Carbs : 0 g Fiber: 0 g Sugar: 0 g Protein: 1 g

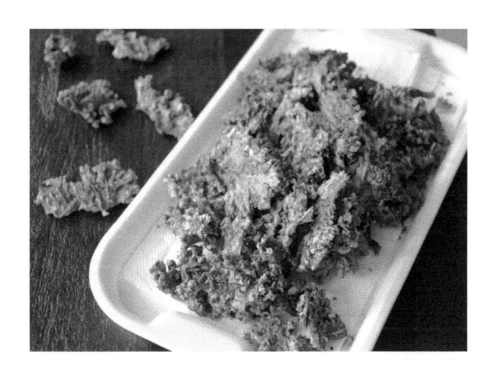

Tasty Hasselback Potatoes
Serves:4

- potatoes wash and dry
- 1 tbsp. Dried thyme
- tbsp. Dried rosemary
- 1 tbsp. Dried parsley
- ½ cup butter, melted
- Pepper
- Salt

Directions:

1.Place potato in hassel back slicer and slice potato using a sharp knife.

2.In a small bowl, mix melted butter, thyme, rosemary, parsley, pepper, and salt.

3.Rub melted butter mixture over potatoes and arrange potatoes on air fryer

4.oven tray.

5.Bake potatoes at 350 f for 25 minutes.

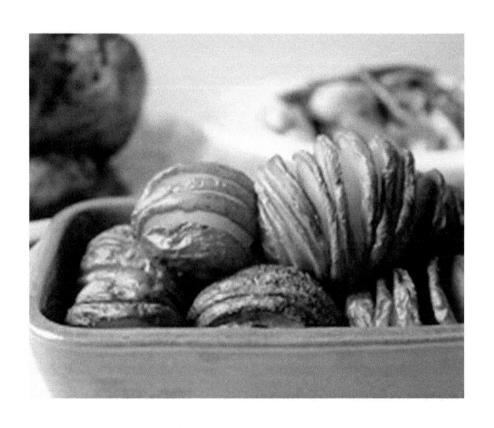

Honey Sriracha Brussels Sprouts

Serves:4

- ½ lb. Brussels sprouts, cut stems then cut each in half
- 1 tbsp. Olive oil
- ½ tsp salt

For Sauce:

- tbsp. Sriracha sauce
- 1 tbsp. Vinegar
- tbsp. Lemon juice –
- 2 tsp Sugar
- 1 tbsp. Honey –
- 1 tsp garlic, minced
- ½ tsp olive oil

Directions:

1.Add all sauce into the small saucepan and heat over low heat for 2-3 minutes or until thickened.

2.Remove saucepan from heat and set aside.

3.Add brussels sprouts, oil, and salt in a zip-lock bag and shake well.

4.Transfer brussels sprouts on air fryer oven tray and air fry at 390 f for 15 minutes. Shake halfway through.

5.Transfer brussels sprouts to the mixing bowl. Drizzle with sauce and toss until well coated.

Roasted Carrots

Serves: 6

- lbs. Carrots, peeled, slice in half again slice half
- 2 ½ tbsp. Dried parsley
- tsp dried oregano
- 1 tsp dried thyme
- 3 tbsp. Olive oil Pepper
- Salt

Directions:

1.Add carrots in a mixing bowl. Add remaining on top of carrots and toss well.

2.Arrange carrots on air fryer oven pan and roast at 400 f for 10 minutes.

3.After 10 minutes turn carrots slices to the other side and roast for 10 minutes more

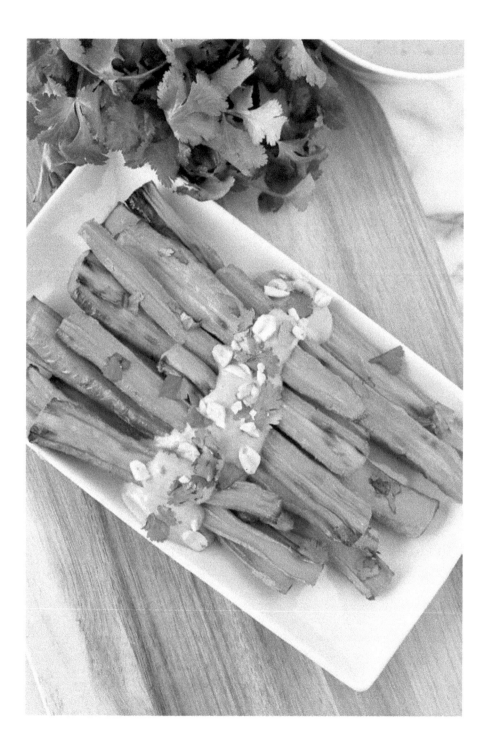

Crunchy Black-Eyed Peas

Servings Provided: 6 **Nutritional Facts Per Serving**:

Protein Count: 9.2 grams Net Carbohydrates: 8.6 grams Total Fat Content: 9.4 grams Calorie Count:262

- Black-eyed peas (15 oz. can)
- Salt (.25 tsp.)
- Chipotle chili powder (.125 tsp.)
- Black pepper (.125 tsp.)
- Chili powder (.5 tsp.)

Directions:

1 Use cold tap water to rinse the beans. Set aside for now.

2 Set the Air Fryer temperature at 360° Fahrenheit.

3 Whisk the spices and add the peas.

4 Add to the fryer basket and air-fry for 10 minutes.

Carrot Mix

Serves: 4

- Coconut milk (2 cups)
- Steel-cut oats (.5 cup)
- Shredded carrots (1 cup)
- Agave nectar (.5 tsp.)
- Ground cardamom (1 tsp.)
- Saffron (1 pinch)

Directions:

1.Lightly spritz the Air Fryer pan using a cooking oil spray.

2.Warm the fryer to reach 365° Fahrenheit.

3.When it's hot, whisk and add the fixings (omit the saffron).

4.Set the timer for 15 minutes.

5.After the timer buzzes, portion into the serving dishes with a sprinkle of saffron.

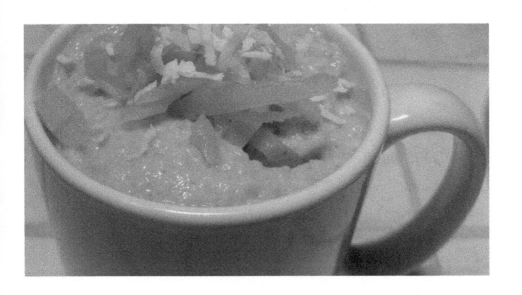

Chinese Breakfast Bowls

Serves:: 4

- Firm tofu (12 oz.)
- Maple syrup (3 tbsp.)
- Coconut aminos (.25 cup)
- Sesame oil (2 tbsp.)
- Lime juice (2 tbsp.)
- Fresh romanesco (1 lb.)
- Carrots (3)
- Red bell pepper (1)
- Cooked red quinoa (2 cups)

Directions:

1. Warm the Air Fryer at 370° Fahrenheit.

2. Cube the tofu and roughly chop the romanesco, carrots, and bell pepper.

3. Combine the juice, aminos, maple syrup, and oil with the tofu cubes in a mixing container.

4. Toss everything into the Air Fryer for 15 minutes. Shake the basket often.

5. Add the peppers, quinoa, spinach, carrots, and romanesco into serving dishes and enjoy.

Easy Breakfast Oats

Serves: 4

- Almond milk (2 cups)
- Steel-cut oats (1 cup)
- Water (2 cups)
- Dried cherries (.33 cup)
- Cocoa powder (2 tbsp.)
- Stevia (.25 cup)
- Almond extract (.5 tsp.)

The Sauce:

- Water (2 tbsp.)
- Cherries (1.5 cups)
- Almond extract (.25 tsp.)

Directions:

Warm the fryer to reach 360° Fahrenheit.

Stir the first set of into the pan of the Air Fryer. Set the timer for 15 minutes.

In a small pot, whisk the sauce fixings. Simmer for 10 minutes.

Portion into serving bowls with a drizzle of the cherry sauce.

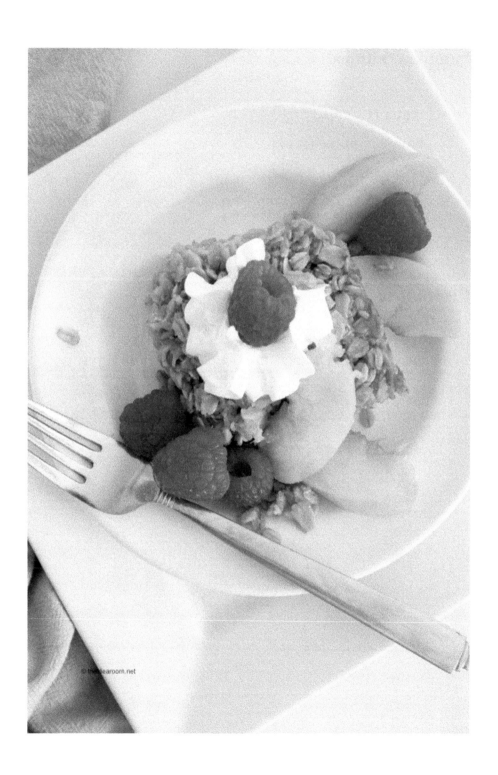

Pumpkin Oatmeal

- Water (1.5 cups)
- Pumpkin puree (.5 cup)
- Stevia (3 tbsp.)
- Pumpkin pie spice (1 tsp.)
- Steel-cut oats (.5 cup)

Directions:

1.Set the Air Fryer at 360° Fahrenheit to preheat.

2.Toss in and mix the fixings into the pan of the Air Fryer.

3.Set the timer for 20 minutes.

4.When the time has elapsed, portion the oatmeal into bowls and serve.

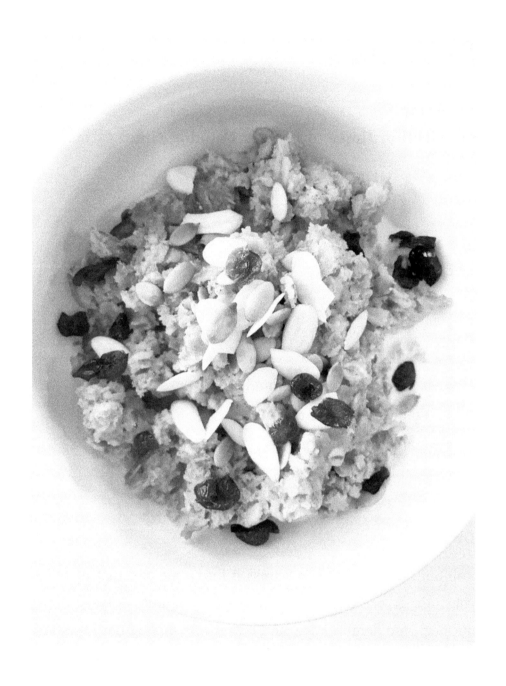

Desserts

Peach Pie

Preparation time: 10 minutes **Cooking time**: 35 minutes
Servings: 4

- 1 pie dough
- 2 and ¼ pounds peaches, pitted and chopped
- 2 tablespoons cornstarch
- ½ cup Sugar
- 2 tablespoons flour
- A pinch of nutmeg, ground
- 1 tablespoon dark rum
- 1 tablespoon lemon juice
- 2 tablespoons butter, melted

Directions:

Roll out the pie dough and press it into a pie pan that matches your air fryer. Combine peaches, cornstarch, sugar, flour, nutmeg, rum, lemon juice, and butter in a mixing bowl and stir well. Pour into a pie pan and spread evenly. Place in your air fryer and cook for 35 minutes at 350 degrees F. Serve warm or cold. Enjoy!

NUTRITION: Calories 231, Fat 6, Fiber 7, Carbs9, Protein 5

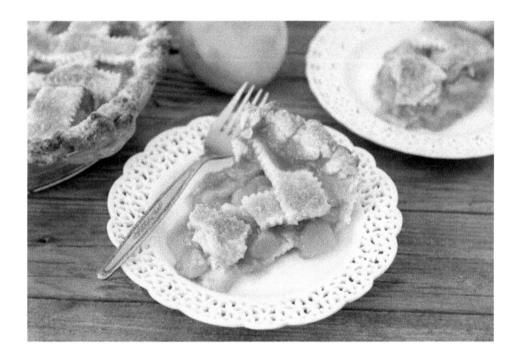

Air Fried Plantains

Servings: 4

- Avocado or sunflower oil (2 tsp.)
- Ripened/almost brown – plantains (2)
- Optional: Salt (.125 tsp.)

Directions:

1.Warm up the Air Fryer to 400° Fahrenheit.

2.Slice the plantains at an angle for a .5-inch thickness.

3.Mix the oil, salt, and plantains in a container – making sure you coat the surface thoroughly.

4.Set the timer for eight to ten minutes; shake after five minutes. If they are not done to your liking, add a minute or two more.

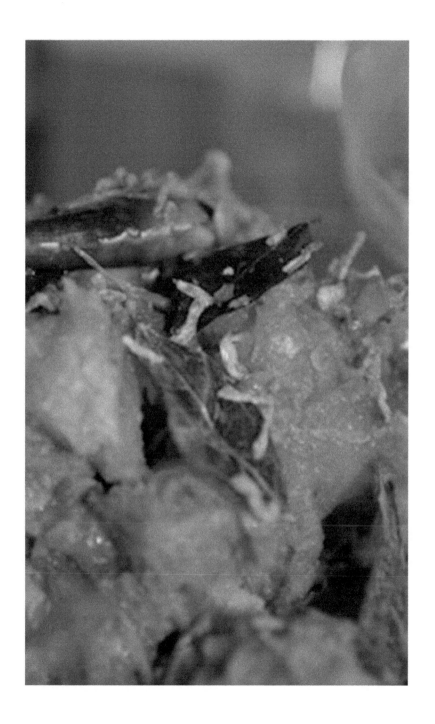

Air Fryer Beignets

Servings: 7

- All-purpose flour (.5 cup)
- White sugar (.25 cup)
- Water (.125 cup)
- Large egg (1 separated)
- Melted butter (1.5 tsp.)
- Baking powder (.5 tsp.)
- Vanilla extract (.5 tsp.)
- Salt (1 pinch)
- Confectioners' sugar (2 tbsp.)
- Also Needed: Silicone egg-bite mold

Directions:

1.Warm the Air Fryer to reach 370° Fahrenheit. Spray the using a nonstick cooking spray.

2.Whisk the flour, sugar, water, egg yolk, butter, baking powder, vanilla extract, and salt together in a large mixing bowl. Stir to combine.

3. Using an electric hand mixer (medium speed), mix the egg white in a small bowl until soft peaks form. Fold into the

4.batter. Pour the mixture into the mold using a small hinged ice cream scoop.

5.Arrange the filled silicone mold in the basket of the Air Fryer.

6.Cook for 10 minutes. Remove mold from the basket carefully, pop the beignets out, and flip them over onto a parchment paper-lined round.

7.Place the parchment round with beignets back into the fryer basket. Cook for another 4 minutes.

8.Remove the beignets from the Air Fryer basket and dust with confectioners' sugar.

9.mold

Banana Smores

Servings: 4

- Bananas (4)
- Mini-peanut butter chips (3 tbsp.)
- Graham cracker cereal (3 tbsp.)
- Mini-semi-sweet chocolate chips (3 tbsp.)

Directions:

1. Heat the Air Fryer in advance to 400° Fahrenheit.
2. Slice the un-peeled bananas lengthwise along the inside of the curve. Don't slice through the bottom of the peel. Open slightly - forming a pocket.
3. Fill each pocket with chocolate chips, peanut butter chips, and marshmallows. Poke the cereal into the filling.
4. Arrange the stuffed bananas in the fryer basket, keeping them upright with the filling facing up.
5. Air-fry until the peel has blackened, and the chocolate and
6. marshmallows have toasted (6 minutes).
7. Cool for 1-2 minutes. Spoon out the filling to serve.

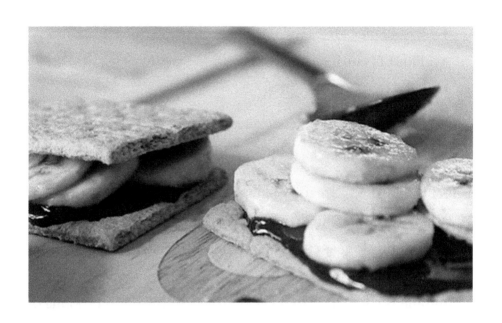

Blackberry & Apricot Crumble

Servings:6

- Fresh blackberries (5.5 oz.)
- Lemon juice (2 tbsp.)
- Fresh apricots (18 oz.)
- Sugar (.5 cup)
- Salt (1 pinch)
- Flour (1 cup)
- Cold butter (5 tbsp.)

Directions:

1.Heat the Air Fryer to 390° Fahrenheit.

2.Lightly grease an 8-inch oven dish with a spritz of cooking oil.

3.Remove the stones, cut the apricots into cubes, and put them in a container.

4.Combine the lemon juice, blackberries, and two tablespoons of sugar with the apricots and mix. Place the fruit in the oven dish.

5.Combine the salt, remainder of the sugar, and flour in a mixing

6.container. Add one tablespoon of cold water and the butter, using your fingertips to make a crumbly mixture.

7.Crumble the mixture over the fruit, pressing them down.

8.Place the dish in the basket and slide it into the Air Fryer. Fry for 20 minutes. It is ready when it is cooked thoroughly, and the top is browned.

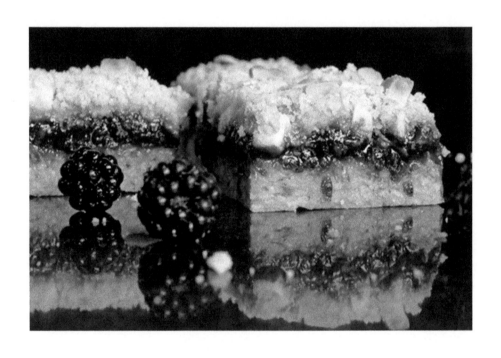